Lions HealthFirst

LIONS

L

INTERNATIONAL

FOUNDATION

Printed in the United States

ISBN: 978-1-387-20281-2

First Publication Date: 1 September 2017

PUBLISHER; LIONS HealthFirst Foundation-USA-NV

3430 E. Flamingo Rd. Las Vegas, NV 89121

101 Tips for a longer, happier and healthier life

From centenarians who have achieved it

By: James Bartel
9/1/2017

"If you want to live to be 100 years old or more and still be healthy, learn from the only true experts, those men and women who've lived it and are role models for all of us".

By: James Bartel, President of the Lions HealthFirst Foundation, a medical charity offering preventative health screenings for seniors from early warning signs of heart disease, stroke and cancer.

The following tips and ideas are from a collection prepared by James Bartel, as Editor of Forever Young, a division of Lions HealthFirst Foundation in Las Vegas Nevada.

Over 30 people ranging in ages from 100 – to – 112 years old shared this information for the benefit of our readers.

INTRODUCTION

The Forever Young concept is a simple one: If you want to live to 100 or more; if you want to be healthy or regain your health, and if you want happiness to surround every aspect of your life, find 100-year-old people who are healthy and happy and discover their secrets.

In 1990, Forever Young's editors began their search for 100-year-old people who've succeeded at mastering life itself. Some are rich and some are poor. Some are highly educated, some are self-educated. Some are business or professional people; some are farmers and factory workers. The one thing they all have in common is longevity and good health.

The fact is; talking to one 100-year-old person about longevity is pure entertainment. But after you've spoken with dozens of these folks, you begin to see amazing consistencies in lifestyle, character, behavior and attitude towards life.

While there's no denying that heredity plays an important role when it comes to health and longevity, it's only one of a number of factors that help determine the quality and quantity of life.

Now, gleaned from dozens of interviews, we bring you the best ideas and advice in this booklet called: **101 Tips for a Healthier, Happier and Longer Life.**

Feel free to pick and choose the ideas most suitable for you. We can't change your lifestyle completely, no one can. But these tips can help bring about small changes that over time can add years to your life, improve your health and help you achieve more happiness.

Attitude Makes the Difference

1) HAVE A REASON FOR LIVING

You must have a reason to get up in the morning, to put your pants on, to remain active. It may be family members that depend on you, career goals, and a pet, even a part-time volunteer job at the local hospital, church or civic organization. The important point is to never stop actively caring about other people.

2) DON'T FIGHT LIFE

Some people complain all the time. Every little aches or pain, every problem, every disappointment is seen as an excuse to moan and groan. The secret to happiness is to accept whatever life offers with a smile and to make the best of whatever situation you're in.

3) DO EVERYTHING IN MODERATION

Moderation is clearly the secret for good health. Don't allow emotions like greed envy or fear to drive you toward excessive behavior. What you eat and drink, how you work and play – all should be done in a sensible way. Maintain a sense of balance in everything you do.

4) TRY SOAKING IN A HOT TUB TO RELAX

World-famous doctor Robert Buckley suggests soaking for 20 minutes or so in a bathtub of warm water with about 40-50 dissolved aspirin. According to Buckley, this safe, simple routine works wonders for all kinds of aches and pains. For a mini-bath, try soaking aching hands or feet for about 15 minutes in a sink or bucketful of warm water with about 10 dissolved aspirin.

5) DEVELOP HEALTHY SELF-ESTEEM

Build confidence and self-esteem by picturing yourself as successful. Working hard at anything – a job, hobby or relationship – can help you develop pride and confidence in yourself and your abilities. Remember, everyone feels frightened and insecure at times. You're not alone. Building up a good sense of self-esteem can help you can cope with the "down" times better.

6) TRY ACTING

Having a bad day? Put on a happy face. Smile, even if it hurts! Before you know it, your whole day will be changed around and life will look pretty good again.

7) PRACTICE GOOD POSTURE

Stand erect, sit straight and learn to move gracefully. You'll look better and feel better about yourself.

8) AVOID FATIGUE

Fatigue rarely comes from overexertion. Under exertion is more likely the cause.

To avoid fatigue:

*Eat well-balanced meals. Don't skimp on breakfast or you'll get tired in the afternoon.

*Exercise more. Exercise increases energy. It also helps you sleep better if you exercise in the early evening.

*Sleep more. If you often get drowsy during the day, go to bed an hour earlier and add an extra hour of sleep at night.

*Work at your peak times. Schedule tough jobs for the time of the day you usually feel most energetic.

*Take breaks. Even if you love your job or the activity you're performing, it helps to stop, stretch, walk or just relax.

9) MEET NEW PEOPLE

If you have a problem getting out meeting new people, try telephoning. Or read the classified ads in the local newspaper. There's usually someone else who's lonely and needs someone to talk to. You might even try running an ad for a companion. Most newspapers will run a "blind ad" box number. Be creative. Let your imagination run amuck. You'll find you're having fun again.

10) DO SOMETHING FOR SOMEONE ELSE

You'll feel better, look better and live longer!

11) COMMUNICATE EFFECTIVELY

Words alone fall upon deaf ears. Most people are so preoccupied with other things that they seldom hear what you're saying. If you want to get someone's attention, you must appeal to one or more of their self-interests – money, romance, self-preservation, and recognition. To accomplish this, try this Emotional Response Techniques (ERT):

*Use words charged with emotional recognition. Words like FIRE have an immediate impact on us. We respond emotionally to anything that threatens our self-preservation or possessions. Words like you, your, our and we all appeal to our desire for recognition.

*Develop mutual respect with the other person. Keep in mind that everyone is looking for respect, recognition and fulfillment.

*Try giving praise. It's one of the best ways to show someone you care. But be sincere about compliments. Use them sparingly and base them upon the person or situation. A false compliment is perceived as a masked insult.

12) RE-ADJUST YOUR "AGING" SETPOINT

You are as old as you feel. Don't worry about the age, those are just numbers.

The key to staying young, according to one gerontologist, is the "aging set point". The set point is ruled by how old you think you are and what you consider middle age. If you're 40 and think you're middle-aged, you're sending a signal to your body to begin to decline. And if you behave and live as if 60 is middle-aged, then you forestall the aging process by telling your body you're only halfway there (human being's potential of 120 years).

13) DON'T ACT OLD

People who age successfully don't act old. They mingle with younger people. They stay as active mentally as they are physically. They look at crisis as a learning experience. They know how to manage stress. They laugh a lot, play and enjoy life. They're optimistic. They see problems as challenges. They're positive.

14) DEVELOP A SOCIAL SUPPORT SYSTEM

People with good social support systems are 2-5 times more likely to outlive those with fewer social involvements. Clearly, having friends is an important element to good mental and physical health. Other pluses include increased adaptability, objectivity, tolerance and open-mindedness. Many people become more productive as they age.

15) GET A PET

Pets can help you live longer. They can cut through depression, anxiety and loneliness and provide a sense of responsibility, usefulness and companionship. And you can get some exercise too when you take your pet outside for its daily walk.

16) LAUGH A LOT

Laughing is good for your health. You may be able to alter your mood favorably with a grin. A good laugh is more than a great tension reliever. It can also aid digestion, lower blood pressure, strengthen muscles, soothe arthritic pain and keep you alert.

17) KEEP YOUR MIND SHARP

Reject the stereotype of helplessness in old age – you'll stay sharper.

Forgetful older people may be the victims of a self-fulfilling prophecy. In fact, recent research suggests that people's ability to make complex judgments and solve problems increases well into their eighties, assuming they stay healthy.

What older people do lose: Abstract reasoning abilities (used in situations such as playing chess). But even here the decline is generally slight and slow.

Who loses the least: People who are socially involved, mentally active and flexible in dealing with new experiences.

18) EXERCISE YOUR MIND

Exercising your mind is important for mental health throughout life. The saying "use it or lose it" applies to the mind as well as the body. One way to get your memory in motion is to get your body moving. Even a 20-30 minute walk three times a week can energize your mind and increase short-term memory, your ability to reason and your reaction time. Although physical exercise is good for both body and mind; there are non-physical activities you can do to stimulate the brain cells such as working crossword puzzles, playing scrabble, trivial pursuit or bridge. These activities will sharpen your memory and increase your ability to recall information.

19) QUIT SMOKING

Cigarette smoking puts you at ten times the risk of getting lung cancer. And it's not just the lungs that are affected. Smoking accounts for approximately 30 percent of all cancer. The pancreas and bladder; for example, are easy targets for cancers that are the result of smoking. Moreover, male smokers develop kidney cancer while female smokers are prone to cervical cancer. There's strong evidence that cigarette smoking causes a host of digestive dysfunctions including heartburn, peptic ulcer (smoking also delays ulcer healing) and esophageal cancer. If you smoke and drink heavily, you are at grave risk of developing cancer of the mouth and throat. And heavy drinkers are at risk of developing cancer of the liver.

Smoking also has a negative effect on taking some medications. Some drugs (for example, Propranolol for heart patients and Tegument for ulcer patients) aren't property metabolized by the liver in smokers.

Now for the good news: As soon as you quit smoking, you decrease your risk of cancer. And your odds get better the longer you're not smoking.

20) KEEP YOUR MEMORY FIT

Older people can practice strategies to reverse memory failure and facilitate learning. Improve concentration by removing yourself from the sights and sounds that distract you. If you're daydreaming, close the curtains. Kids clamoring about? Close the door. Talk yourself through tasks to focus attention. Establish a "memory place" in the house where you put things like glasses, keys and mail. Notes and calendars are good reminders.

21) PRE-PLAN YOUR RETIREMENT

Pre-Retirement counselors can help you make sense of health benefits, pension plans, IRA's, social security, etc. Practice your next vacation as a trail retirement; develop new interests, new routines. Renegotiate roles with your spouse and discuss what you both have in mind regarding use of leisure time, retirement finances, etc. If you are thinking of moving after retirement, try visiting the location for extended periods first.

LEARN HOW TO HANDLE STRESS

Everyone must face stressful situations on a regular basis. How you handle them can make the difference between a having healthy mind and body, or disease. Here are some tips on how to handle stress.

22) DON'T TAKE YOURSELF TOO SERIOUSLY

Take time out to laugh and enjoy life. Care about someone or something other than yourself.

23) KEEP ACTIVE

Exercise, dance, go to the mall – do anything to exercise your mind and body. Don't wait for the doorbell to ring – go out and make social contacts. Build up routines that include time to work, play, socialize and be alone. Develop goals that keep you wanting to get up every morning.

24) LEARN TO SAY NO

Don't always be so nice. A lot of people suffering from stress are doing too many things to be nice or because they can't say no.

25) TAKE TIME OUT FOR YOURSELF

A 20 minute soak in a hot bath, a long walk, reading a book, even talking with a friend, can help reduce stress.

26) GET A HOBBY – HAVE SOME FUN

Set aside part of the day for having fun. Do at least one thing you enjoy each day.

27) SET GOALS

Keep a diary and list what you want to achieve now and in the long-run. Goal-setting helps define priorities and gives you a sense of self-control – a key weapon against stress.

28) LEARN HOW TO RELAX

Use meditation, deep breathing or some other form of relaxation to reduce blood pressure and relax muscles. Regular practice of some type of relaxation method can help develop your resistance to stress.

29) TRY MEDITATING

Meditating rejuvenates the mind and body. It starts with deep muscle relaxation. As physical stress melts away, the mind begins to unwind and negative emotions are released.

30) START CARING FOR SOMETHING

Caring has a lot to do with mental health. Whether it's a pet, a garden, a house or other people; you're protecting yourself from self-despair when you care for something.

31) LEARN TO LET OFF STEAM

Stress doesn't make you sick, but the way you handle it may. Several studies suggest that how you react to stressful events like the death of a loved one; or retirement can affect your immune system and leave you more susceptible to diseases, including cancer.

32) SEEK EMOTIONAL SUPPORT FROM FRIENDS

People in tense situations have a less harmful physical response when in the presence of a friend. Emotional support provided by the presence of a friend or companion can make the situation less stressful for the heart.

33) PRACTIVE COPING SKILLS FOR A LIFETIME

There is evidence that those who cope the most positively with stress consider it natural for things to change. They anticipate change as a useful stimulus to development. Consequently, they suffer less from psychological signs of stress.

34) AVOID BOREDOM

Boredom can cause as much personal stress as pressure does, and the effects may be even worse. Drug addiction, for example, can often be traced to boredom. The best way to avoid boredom is to always be learning something new and planning something to look forward to.

Helpful hint: Wean yourself from mental opiates such as soap operas and pulp fiction.

THE IMPORTANCE OF SLEEP

Sleep refreshes the mind and body. It's a prime time for healing and tissue renewal, since it's the time when cell division and protein synthesis are fastest and the body's immune system is at its most efficient. Sleep also appears to aid memory. Many of the above tips on stress will help you get a good night sleep. Here are some other tips as well.

35) RECOGNIZE AND ACCEPT INDIVIDUAL SLEEPING PATTERNS

Some people do fine on four hours of sleep, some needs ten. Remember, as you get older, you may require less sleep. Increased daytime drowsiness, lighter sleep and frequent awakenings during the night are all common in older people. But overall, your sleep shouldn't change much as you age.

36) DRINK A WARM GLASS OF MILK

Warm milk contains an amino acid called L-tryptophan that has been shown to stimulate a brain compound called serotonin, which may fight depression, kill pain and aid asleep. Cheddar cheese, peanuts, turkey, tuna are also good sources of L-tryptophan. L-tryptophan tablets are also available. Consult your doctor before taking the tablets though, because they don't work for everyone.

Eating foods high in complex carbohydrates releases insulin that in turn helps clear the way for L-tryptophan to be carried to the brain.

37) DON'T EAT TOO MUCH OR TOO LITTLE BEFORE BEDTIME

Digesting a large meal stimulates the body, lightens sleep and arouses the sleeper. Eating too little leads to knowing hunger pains that can cause restlessness and a poor night's sleep. Try eating a banana with a glass of milk or even a small tuna sandwich if you're hungry right before bedtime.

38) REVIEW ALL DRUGS AND MEDICATIONS

Nicotine and caffeine in your body can increase the amount of time it takes you to fall asleep.

The main ingredient in over-the-counter sleeping pills is actually an antihistamine, which may produce some potentially serious side effects if used for prolonged periods. It can cause glaucoma to worsen, produce irregular heartbeats and urinary problems. Antibiotics, or any prescription, may also disturb sleep. Check with your doctor or pharmacist if you experience any sleep disturbances while taking medications.

And forget that "nightcap" – it can ruin your night. Although alcohol initially induces sleepiness, after two or three hours it arouses your nervous system to higher level than before and you actually become more awake and restless.

39) REFINE YOUR SLEEP ROUTINE

Your body functions on a normal circadian rhythm (your "body clock") that tells it when and how much sleeps it needs. Develop a normal sleep routine in-sync with your body's own natural rhythm.

*Don't Go To Bed Until You're Sleepy. Do something relaxing until you feel tired.

*Develop Your Own Sleep Rituals. Close all the windows, lock the doors, wash up, read a book. Sleep rituals prepare you psychologically as well as physically for sleep.

40) KEEP YOUR WAKE-UP TIME CONSISTENT

Get up at the same time every day regardless of what time you go to sleep. This accomplishes two things: It resets the body's circadian rhythm so that it expects to get up from sleep at the same time tomorrow, and it synchronizes all other sleep and wake cycles.

Also, if you take a nap during the day, follow a regular schedule. Keep it short – about 30 minutes – and plan it for late in the morning or early afternoon.

40) GET SOME EXERCISE DURING THE DAY

You'll fall asleep easier and sleep better if you get some exercise during the day. But do it in the late afternoon or early evening since strenuous exercise can stimulate the cardiovascular and nervous system for hours, making it difficult for you to relax. And exercise in moderation.

41) INCREASE YOUR MENTAL ACTIVITY

Isolation, boredom and lack of social contacts can all disrupt sleep. Get involved in a project or do volunteer work. Do something to keep your mind active and stimulated.

42) INCREASE YOUR MENTAL ACTIVITY

Isolation, boredom and lack of social contacts can all disrupt sleep. Get involved in a project or do volunteer work. Do something to keep your mind active and stimulated.

DOCTORS AND MEDICATION

43) TAKE AN ACTIVE, INFORMED ROLE IN YOUR MEDICAL CARE

Don't underestimate the importance of your relationship with your doctor. If you aren't comfortable with your physician and can't exchange information in a down-to-earth way, you may not feel comfortable about following his or her advice. Moreover, having faith in your doctor may be a factor in whether you heal or not; treatment is more likely to be successful if you have a great deal of faith in your physician's ability.

44) BECOME THE MASTER OF YOUR MEDICATIONS

Make sure your doctor offers you information about drugs he prescribes. When your physician pulls out the prescription pad, you pull out your list of questions. At the top of the list should be the question "Is this drug necessary?" In other words, ask as diplomatically as you can if there might be non-drug approaches. This question is especially important to ask if psychoactive drugs (those that affect the mind or behavior) are prescribed.

45) CUT DOWN ON MEDICATIONS

People over 65 take about three times the number of prescription drugs than those under 65. Before you take medication for an ache or pain, see if there is natural cure that doesn't require medication.

Doctor has a tendency to over-medicate older patients. Mind altering drugs are often given in an attempt to relieve the effects of such life problems as isolation, loneliness or loss. Instead of automatically considering drugs as the only option, make social contacts or develop new interests whenever possible.

46) USE OVER-THE-COUNTER MEDICINES WISELY

This is especially important if you take other drugs. Consult your pharmacist and read labels. Look for hidden ingredients you can do without. Some aspirin preparations contain caffeine, and cough medicine frequently contains alcohol.

47) LEARN THE WARNING SIGNS

Stop taking a drug if you experience confusion, difficulty in urination, dry mouth, blurry vision or any other symptom which started after you began taking the drug.

48) FOLLOW DIRECTIONS

That means take all your medications. Sounds basic enough, yet it's surprising how many people stop taking pills like antibiotics at the first inkling of recovery. The trouble with this is that the bug could return and hit you with a bigger bout than ever. You may also get yourself in trouble with the opposite kind of thinking: "If one pill makes me feel good, two pills will make me feel great." Wrong. Overdosing makes you feel worse. Remember, too, that pills are personalized, so don't exchange them with your friends. And don't hoard them "just in case" either. Drugs are only guaranteed to be potent up to the expiration date – using them after that time could be dangerous if their chemical composition has changed.

49) STICK TO A SCHEDULE

Set up a system that helps you remember to take your medicine. Whatever the system, be sure to explain it to someone else – just in case. There are many methods available for addressing the problem of medication mix-ups – pills may come pre-arranged according to dosage time and days, much the same way most oral contraceptives are packaged, or you can buy pill dispensers with separate compartments for days of the week.

50) LEARN TO MAKE THE MEDICINE GO DOWN

Unless otherwise directed, your best bet is to take medications with nothing but plain water – a whole glassful, at that. That way our make sure the drug gets into your bloodstream and does what it's supposed to do. From the American Medical Association comes a tip for taking tablets: Put a little water in your mouth and tilt your head back. Tilt your head forward when swallowing capsules. Don't take pills while lying down – they may dissolve in the esophagus and cause heartburn, nausea or vomiting.

51) BEWARE OF DRUG INTERACTIONS

One drug may cancel out another or magnify its potency. Over-the –counter antacids can block the body's ability to absorb medicines, including some antibiotics. Even aspirin can cause problems because it can intensify the effects of some medications, including blood thinners. Keep a list of all the drugs you take – prescriptions and over-the –counter – in your wallet or pocket-book and give your pharmacists a copy of the list.

52) TAKE SLEEPING PILLS WITH CAUTION

Long-acting sleeping pills generally do their work and pass through the body within 18 hours. But as you get older, ingredients may remain active for up to three or four days. This can result in confusion and forgetfulness, even depression.

Most over-the-counter sleeping pills are merely antihistamines, which may cause serious side effects if used for prolonged periods of time. (See hint #36)

53) DON'T DRINK WHILE TAKING DRUGS

You're asking for a double dose of drowsiness or even more if you combine alcohol with medications such as antihistamines, insulin, high blood pressure drugs, antibiotics and tranquilizers. The problem may be more pronounced as you age since alcohol stays in the bloodstream longer.

54) AVOID SMOKING WITH CERTAIN DRUGS

You should also say no to nicotine if you take medications. Smoking can cancel out the effects of some drugs.

55) DON'T BE MISLED BY MIRACULOUS CLAIMS

This is particularly true when considering claims for drugs which supposedly extend life or reverse the damage done by aging. Because the aging process is so complex, it is very unlikely that a single nutrient, hormone or techniques will ever stop or reverse all the changes. Use caution in assessing any claim for a life-extending or rejuvenating agent.

LEARNING TO DEAL WITH GRIEF AS A NORMAL LIFE EXPERIENCE

Grief is the most profound emotion you'll ever experience. It can wreak havoc on your immune system and leave you vulnerable to a variety of physical ailments. Here are some tips on how to deal effectively with grief and loss.

56) PREPARE FOR LOSS

How you deal with grief depends to a large extent upon your perspective and preparedness to deal with loss. Fear, not grief, is often the culprit. Don't let fears of death (yours or that of a loved one) immobilize you to the point that you deny your grief. Denial can lead to chronic disorientation. Develop adaption skills before you face a major loss.

57) DISCUSS ANTICIPATED CHANGES

You can prepare for more serious setbacks if you think about them honestly and plan what to do. One way to prepare is to talk about it beforehand. Frank discussion about emotions, as well as resources such as finances, etc., can help you prepare.

58) PRACTICE GRIEVING SKILLS DAILY

Look at life as an opportunity to practice grieving skills on a daily basis and you can better prepare for the more serious setbacks. Missing an appointment, getting stood-up by a date, facing financial setbacks or loss of independence – these daily losses offer you the opportunity to practice grieving skills. Learn to deal with the anger, rage, guilt, impatience and acceptance of these losses as a preview of the way you'll handle the major losses.

59) LEARN THE STAGES OF DYING – AND LIVING

The five stages of dying are denial, anger, bargaining, depression, and acceptance. They're also the five stages of living. Be aware of these stages when facing small daily losses and grief will become a healthy, natural part of living.

60) HONOR YOUR FEELINGS

Sorrow, guilt, anger, depression, loneliness, fear, anxiety, and shame are all normal emotions associated with bereavement. Don't be afraid to voice these emotions openly and honestly. By telling your story to family and friends over and over, you clarify in your mind what has happened and how you really feel about it, and you learn to accept the reality of the loss.

61) TRY A HEALTHY CRY

Crying can provide a healthy outlet. Tears carry away toxins that are produced during emotional shocks and can relieve tension and stress.

62) SEEK A NURTURING SOCIAL NETWORK

Mourners who have the support of family and friends fare much better than those who don't. Surround yourself with loved ones who can support you through the grieving stages.

63) EAT RIGHT

With the added stress of grieving, it's important to stay physically healthy. Make sure that your eating habits remain stable. Don't eat too much or too little. Choose nutritious foods and make sure you drink plenty of caffeine-free and alcohol-free beverages.

64) GET PLENTY OF REST

Rest when you feel the urge and maintain normal sleeping patterns. Don't push yourself to keep busy or preoccupied at all times. Grief isn't something you can run away from. Rest and solitude are regenerative.

YOU ARE WHAT YOU EAT

65) EAT A BALANCED DIET

Foods you should be eating include cholesterol fighters, fiber foods rich in gums (oatmeal and dried beans) and pectin (citrus fruits, cabbage, carrots, etc). These fibers bind to the bile acids that digest fats and remove them from the body. Also, when gums and pectin coat the stomach it slows sugar absorption which is a bonus to diabetics.

66) EAT HIGH PROTEIN MEALS

People who eat a high-carbohydrate meal are sleepier two hours later than those who have eaten a high-protein meal.

67) EAT LESS SUGAR

Sugar is tougher on your body as you grow older. Healthy people ages 22 – 30 have twice the insulin-binding abilities of people 40 – 59. Older people become more glucose-intolerant.

68) CHOOSE FOODS TO LOWER BLOOD PRESSURE

Here are some basic guidelines to help you select healthy foods:

- o Eat Less Salt.
- o Eat Less Fat. While you're avoiding the saltshaker, you might try snubbing the butter, bacon and cheese too.
- o Drink Less Alcohol. So far, medical evidence indicates that drinking more than three beers, three glasses of wine or three mixed drinks (one ounce of alcohol each) per day can indeed raise blood pressure.

o Eat More Food With Potassium. Cantaloupe, winter squash, avocados, orange juice, bananas, potatoes, tomatoes, and milk are all good choices.

o Eat Food High in Calcium. You'll find this mineral in dairy products, leafy green vegetables and beans.

o Get More Magnesium. This mineral is found in nuts, brown rice, molasses, milk, wheat germ, bananas, potatoes and soy products.

o Eat More Fish. Especially haddock, mackerels, sardines, trout, and salmon.

o Eat More Fiber. Be sure to eat plenty of fresh fruit and vegetables, beans and whole-grain breads, as well as bran.

69) EAT FOOD HIGH IN FIBER

The foods that add fiber to your diet include far more than just bran and whole grains. Even more valuable sources of fiber are beans, other vegetables and fruits.

Best alternatives in Vegetables: Peas, potatoes, okra, broccoli, zucchini, summer squash.

In Beans: Kidney, white, black and pinto.

In Fruits: Apples, blackberries, pears, and strawberry.

Other High Fiber Foods: Popcorn, sesame seeds.

70) EAT HIGH-FIBER AND HIGH-CALCIUM FOODS AT DIFFERENT TIMES

Fiber can prevent the body from absorbing calcium.

71) DON'T GET CARRIED AWAY WITH BRAN

Excessive amounts of bran can strip the body of iron since bran often unites with iron. Iron is thus carried through the body without being absorbed.

72) AVOID DANGEROUS DIETS

Avoid weight-loss programs that:

- Promise rapid weight loss (more than 1% of total body weight per week).

- Make you dependent on special products rather than teach you how to make good choices from conventional foods.
- Do not encourage permanent, realistic lifestyle changes.
- Misrepresent salespeople as "counselors" supposedly qualified to give guidance in nutrition and/or general health.
- Require a large sum of money at the start, or require you to sign a contract for an expensive, long-term program.
- Fail to inform you about the various health risks associated with weight loss.
- Promote unproven weight-loss aids.
- Claim that 'cellulite' exists in the body.
- Claim that the use of an appetite suppressant or bulking agent enables you to lose fat without restricting caloric intake.
- Claim that a weight-control product contains a unique ingredient or component, unless that component really is not available in other weight-loss products.

73) EAT LARGER MEALS EARLY IN THE DAY

Diets work better when you eat more of your food early in the day. Calories consumed early in the day are more likely to be converted to energy rather than stored as fat.

74) DRINK TEA (IN MODERATION) FOR ITS BENEFITS

Tea mimics antidepressant drugs. Its caffeine helps the brain synthesize chemical stimulants, then, its polyphenols help keep those chemicals in the body longer.

Unlike coffee, tea does not raise blood cholesterol levels. It actually strengthens blood-vessel walls and may even cut cholesterol absorption.

Rich in fluoride, tea inhibits growth of decay-causing bacteria in dental plaque.

It's a good source of zinc, manganese and potassium, and its tannin helps preserve Vitamin C in the body.

Hot tea fights colds by doubling mucus flow, which helps to wash out germs.

Herbal teas on the other hand can be dangerous because they sometimes counter the effects of prescription drugs or cause serious side effects like severe diarrhea, allergic reactions, toxic reactions, and hallucinations.

75) REDUCE CAFFEINE INTAKE

Caffeine taken in excess is associated with heart irritation and an approximately 10% rise in serum cholesterol levels.

Two to three cups of caffeinated beverages can raise blood pressure significantly, especially in those over 50.

Too much caffeine can also cause a loss of calcium and magnesium from the body. This presents a particular threat to women who need the extra calcium to prevent osteoporosis.

Caffeine can also interfere with some drugs effects. Example: Since caffeine reduces the body's iron absorption, it is inadvisable to drink caffeinated beverages within two hours of taking an iron pill.

76) DRINK PLENTY OF WATER

Aging bodies needs at least six glasses of water every day.
Reason: A young adult's body is 60% water, but this amount decreases with age. Result: Skin dries out and the kidneys don't flush wastes as well. Drinking more water keeps skin from becoming dry. And water dilutes salt and minerals that pass through the kidneys helping prevent kidney stones.

GETTING THE MOST FROM VITAMINS

77) STORE VITAMINS EFFECTIVELY

Don't refrigerate vitamins. The supplements will collect moisture, causing them to lose their potency. And because it absorbs moisture, always remove the cotton that comes in the bottle. Store vitamins and minerals in a cool, dark, dry place; such as a cupboard away from the stove.

78) GET VITAMINS INTO YOUR SYSTEM THE FASTEST WAY

Contrary to popular belief, timed-released vitamin supplements are the least well-absorbed by the body. Best absorbed: Vitamin solutions, followed by chewable tablets and conventional tablets.

79) EXERCISE REGULARLY SO VITAMINS WORK

Vitamins may work best when supplemented by regular exercise. When two groups were given daily doses of Vitamins C and E for two months, there was little change in the immune system of the sedentary people. The exercisers, however, experienced a significant increase in immunity.

80) PREVENT FADING MEMORY

Short-term memory tends to fade as you age. But you can stay sharper longer by avoiding vitamin deficiencies (particularly B12) ... limiting yourself to no more than two alcoholic drinks a day ... keeping your blood pressure down ... and staying mentally active through reading, writing, crosswords puzzles, etc.

81) BEWARE OF VITAMIN DEPLETERS

Smoking: Drains up to 40% of Vitamin C supplies.

Alcohol: B1, B6, B12, and C.

Steroids: Calcium.

Antibiotics and oral contraceptives: B Vitamins.

Strict vegetarianism: B12.

82) TAKE CALCIUM CORRECTLY

Calcium supplements won't work if taken under the wrong conditions. Calcium carbonate (the most common supplement) is absorbed by an empty stomach only in the presence of stomach acid. But in many older people, gastric acids may diminish or even shut off entirely. So always take calcium carbonate with a meal.

Calcium supplements are best absorbed in small amounts and should be spaced throughout the day. They are best taken at bedtime; skeletal calcium tends to be drawn on more at night when no food is being eaten. For maximum absorption, have a glass of milk or some yogurt before taking the supplement.

83) DON'T OVERDOSE

The old advice is still the best – there is no reason to take more than the recommended dietary allowance (RDA) of any vitamin except for relatively rare individuals who cannot absorb or utilize vitamins adequately.

A mega dose is 10 or more times the RDA. This is the level at which toxic effects begin to show up in adults. Even in cases of actual vitamin insufficiency, mega doses are not generally prescribed. Therapeutic doses are generally smaller than 10 times the RDA.

For people who don't eat properly or want nutritional insurance, take a regular multivitamin capsule containing only the RDA of vitamins.

84) LEARN THE FACTS ABOUT VITAMIN C
- *Don't take Vitamin C and Aspirin at the same time.*

Vitamin C and aspirin should not be taken together. Studies indicate that combined heavy doses produce excessive stomach irritation that could lead to ulcers (especially for those with a history of stomach problems).

- *Vitamin C and Aging.*

Doctors now believe that Vitamin C may help slow the aging process. Vitamin C seems to combat oxidation (considered by many the basis of aging) at the cellular level. Note: Vitamin E also retards the aging process, but unlike Vitamin C, it can be harmful if taken in excess.

- *Beware of chewable Vitamin C.*

Chewing the vitamin creates an acid imbalance in the mouth that erodes tooth enamel, particularly in the rear of the mouth. Excessive Vitamin C in some fruit juices can create the same situation.

85) AVOID ZINC DEFICIENCY

Zinc is crucial for a strong immune system. Zinc deficiency tends to worsen with age. An early warning sign of zinc deficiency is when food starts to taste bland. So protect against infection and put some zest back into your food by making sure you get the RDA of 15 – 30mg a day.

86) ABSORB IRON FROM YOUR FOOD

The iron in food is absorbed better when you eat foods rich in vitamin C at the same meal.

Iron Blockers: Tea, antacids and dietary fiber supplements.

EXERCISE – STILL ONE OF THE BEST PREVENTATIVE MEDICINES

Regular physical exercise, extolled for its healthful effects on the heart and circulatory system, is now believed to help delay the aging process. Once thought to add wear and tear to the body, vigorous physical activity has been shown to improve body tissue and functions. Some benefits of aerobic activity that slow down aging: More energy, less depression and anxiety; better digestion, stronger bones, reduced cardiovascular diseases.

87) WALK FOR BETTER HEALTH

Walking is the safest way for anyone, at any age, to begin exercising since you can start slowly and build up speed and distance with minimal risk. It's an inexpensive, safe and sociable way to keep fit. Walking can be every bit as much as aerobic exercise as more strenuous sports. If done properly and at a brisk rate, it can strengthen the heart and lungs. A sustained, vigorous walk can strengthen muscles and build tone, increase endurance, aid in digestion and elimination, relieve tension and help in weight control.

88) DANCE, DANCE, DANCE

Dancing offers an excellent, gentle, low-impact aerobic workout. Unlike other forms of aerobic exercise, dancing is one almost anyone can do without risk of injury.

When followed over a period of time, a vigorous dance program results in the same benefits as any aerobic exercise program: loss of body fat, increased muscle tone, slowing of the aging process, improved stamina and endurance, increased energy and resistance to fatigue, and improved efficiency of the heart and lung functions.

Regular dancing also improves posture, coordination, balance and flexibility. And, it does wonders for your social life too!

89) DO IT RIGHT

Correct breathing and posture during exercise are essential. Even basic exercises done improperly can cause or aggravate injuries.

- o Toe touching: Doing this with the knee in a locked position and with a rapid bouncing action places tremendous pressure on the lumbar vertebrae which could result in lower back pains. Allow your knees to bend slightly, and remain in a hanging-over position for three complete slow deep breaths. Then straighten slowly. Repeat this three times slowly. Do it without bouncing.
- o Leg lifts: Performing these while lying on your back and raising both legs at the same time can cause the pelvis to rotate and lead to swayback (the problem of lower back lordosis). Eliminate this exercise altogether.
- o Sit-ups: Doing these with straight legs can also contribute to an increase curvature of the lower back. For the abdominal muscles to get a real workout, bend your knees, keep your feet flat on the floor, fold your arms over your chest, and curl up to only a 30 degree angle from the floor.
- o Deep knee bends: These can cause injury to knee cartilage. Bending the knees so that they are directly over the feet and the thighs are parallel to the floor will not cause injury.

90) AVOID SPORADIC WORKOUTS

Regular, moderate exercise is more healthful than more intensive but sporadic workouts. A person lowers "bad" cholesterol and raises "good" cholesterol in proportion to the time spent in physical activity. But high intensity exercise by itself has no effect. Bottom line: A brisk walk or slow jog for 30 minutes a day is better than a heavy weekend workout.

91) EXERCISE TO FIGHT FATIGUE

Exercise is a better way to fight late-afternoon fatigue than the traditional cup of coffee, soft drink or cigarette. These can leave you feeling just as groggy an hour later. A brief walk or several jumping jacks does a better job of waking up the body. Eating the right food earlier in the day also helps – protein for breakfast and a light lunch.

92) BEWARE OF DRUGS' EFFECTS WHEN EXERCISING

Drugs and exercise can be a hazardous combination. Aspirin can mask the pain that should tell you to stop. Antihistamines can cause drowsiness and strain the heart and muscles. Decongestants raise overall blood pressure. Diuretics can lead to dehydration and cramping. Tranquilizers, besides robbing you of your competitive edge, dull your perception of pain. Best advice: take a new drug at least twice and gauge your reaction before adding the stress of exercise. And never combine multiple drugs with exercise without consulting your doctor.

93) STICK WITH IT

The average exercise or diet regimen lasts only four days. Before you start one, imagine yourself doing it regularly and for the long haul.
Exercise layoffs quickly erode gains made in heart and lung capacity. The steepest drop is during the first 12 days of inactivity. After that, the fitness decline continues at a slower rate. Advice: after suspending exercise because of illness or other reasons, resume your workout at a lower level to give your body time to work back up.

94) TRY PASSIVE EXERCISES

Vigorous exercise isn't the only way to stay healthy. An easier way to help circulation and relax your nervous system: Lie on your back on the floor. Raise your lower legs and rest them on a chair, with knees relaxed and slightly bent. Keep them there for five to ten minutes. Do this once or twice a day.

95) TRY NATURAL EXERCISE

If you hate formal exercise, you can still stay fit through natural activity. Walk for 20 minutes a day in loose-fitting clothes and soft shoes. Try the "M&M" policy: Move More. Take the stairs instead of elevators. Walk for the paper. Stow your golf cart and carry your own bag.

96) EXERCISE AFTER EATING

Working off a big meal is easier than you think. Exercising soon after eating is an efficient way to burn excess calories. Reason: Since both eating a good meal and exercising raise your body's metabolic rate, you use up more calories exercising after a meal than before one. (Conversely, cutting back on calories lowers your metabolism and makes you work harder to burn off what you eat). Minimum requirement for working off a meal: A 20-minute walk and 45-minutes of eating.

97) EAT A BANANA FOR A PRE-WORKOUT SNACK

A banana is an ideal pre-workout snack. It's easily digested and converted rapidly into energy. It compensates for body losses of potassium. And a single banana provides 20% of the RDA of Vitamin B6 (essential for building muscle tissues).

98) DRINK PLENTY OF WATER DURING EXERCISE

For top athletic performance, make sure your body gets enough water. Guidelines: Drink two cups of water 15 minutes before exercise or competition ... one cup every 15-30 minutes during the activity ... and at least two cups beyond thirst requirements when activity is over. Sports drinks, which contain sugar and salt, take longer to reach the blood-stream than pure water.

99) WARM-UP BEFORE EXERCISING

Myth: Stretching is the best way to warm up before exercising.

Reality: Stretching doesn't generate enough heat to warm up muscles.

It's better to start the activity at a slower rate. Take a fast walk before you run ... toss a ball easily before throwing it hard. (Stretching, however, has its own value in keeping muscles flexible).

100)   SWIM FOR A GREAT OVERALL WORKOUT

Swimming helps the entire musculature of the body, particularly the upper torso. It tones muscles, but doesn't build them.

Greatest benefit: The cardiovascular system.

101) WALK TALL TO PREVENT FORGETFULNESS, KEEP YOUR MIND YOUNG

Paying attention to your posture is a good way to keep your brain performing at its peak. Allowing your upper body to sag, with rounded shoulders, head hung over and chin jutting outward, can create kinks in the spine that squeeze the two arteries passing through the spinal column to the brain. This causes an inadequate blood supply which results in fuzzy thinking and forgetfulness, especially as you age. So walk tall – keep your head back and your chin in.

These are some of the most powerful, yet simple tools and techniques for relieving stress, living a happier and healthier life, and living to your full potential.